# 1 Patients in pain

It is now almost ten years since a joint working party of the Royal College of Surgeons and the College of Anaesthetists reported that 'the treatment of pain after surgery in British hospitals has been inadequate and has not advanced significantly for years'. (Ref. 2). Four years after that report, a large-scale survey of patients in hospital found that of 3,000 patients, nine out of ten had been in moderate or severe pain at some point, and three out of ten said that the pain had been present all or most of the time (Ref. 3). The Audit Commission further found that some hospitals – and some wards – are better than others at controlling pain, even when casemix is taken into account (Ref. 1). The number of patients reporting pain after their daycase hernia operation, for example, differs significantly between hospitals **[EXHIBIT 1, overleaf].**

The experience of unrelieved post-operative pain can lead to high levels of dissatisfaction among patients, a slower recovery, and even complications:

- acute pain may affect respiratory function, which may lead to a chest infection and respiratory failure;

- patients in pain are less easily mobilised and so there is an increased likelihood of deep vein thrombosis and pulmonary embolism;

EXHIBIT 1

Some hospitals are better than others at controlling pain, even when casemix is taken into account.

*Source: Database of 11,053 day surgery patients operated on in 43 hospitals between 1991 and 1995 (only the hospitals with more than 10 hernia patients are plotted; see Audit Commission [Ref.1] for more details.)*

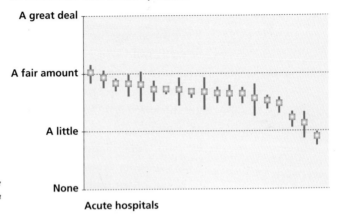

**Pain reported by patients during the 24 hours after their hernia operation**

• pain is a significant risk factor in the development of pressure sores; and

• older people sometimes get confused as a result of pain and some painkillers.

The popular assumption that serious pain after surgery is unavoidable is misplaced. With good collaboration between nurses, anaesthetists, surgeons, and pharmacists, patients can expect post-operative pain to be well-managed and kept to acceptable levels.

Patients do not always get effective pain relief for a variety of reasons:

1 **Effective pain relief is not achieved** – either because the doctors have not prescribed adequate analgesics, because trainee doctors and nurses administer less

than the prescribed dose, or because the regimen is not tailored to the patient's individual needs.

Ward staff may administer less than the prescribed dose because they mistakenly believe that administering repeated doses of morphine to patients in pain risks addiction or because they are working to traditional (and outmoded) routines, such as 'three doses of post-operative opiates and then on to paracetamol' or 'morphine every four hours'. Attitudes and responses to pain such as these effectively hinder a good pain relief service.

2  **Patients do not tell staff that they are in pain –** because they do not know how much pain it is reasonable to expect and are not sure when and if to tell someone about their pain. A great many worry about 'making a fuss' and feel that it is usually best to 'grin and bear it'. In extreme cases, patients wait unitl they are in severe pain before they complain.

*'There's not always something they can do.'*
Interviewed patient

3  **Nurses underestimate patients' experience of pain –** although nurses are responsible for assessing and relieving patients' pain, they often underestimate the severity of that pain and do not always use objective tools to assess pain (Ref. 4).

*'Some nurses understand [how bad the pain is] more than others.'* Interviewed patient

4   **There is a delay in administering pain relief** – and
pain is less easy to control once it has been allowed
to break through. Patients sometimes wait until they
are in a great deal of pain before they ask for pain
relief, and then that delay is followed by a further
delay in administering the analgesics which take time
to take effect. Analgesics should always be provided
before procedures involving potentially painful
movement (washing, getting out of bed) – walking
is particularly difficult if a patient is in pain.

*'[My request] was not dealt with quickly... It can take
one and a half hours to get back so you wait in pain.'*
Interviewed patient

*'I call the nurse if the pain [near the operation site]
is severe, otherwise they come round with the drug
trolley. You wait for the drug round to finish and
they bring something to you.'* Interviewed patient

5   **Pain relief is not monitored** – and ward staff fail
to check how a patient has responded to pain relief.
Only by finding out if a dose is effective can further
doses be adjusted to suit the patient. Patients may
also suffer if nurses do not record and exchange
information about the success or failure of different
measures – something they should do using written
plans and evaluations.

*'Some tablets are better than others. The pain never
goes away.'* Interviewed patient

# 2

## Information for patients

Information given to patients about what to expect can reduce post-operative pain and anxiety (Ref. 1). But patients do not always get enough information either about pain itself or about pain relief, and sometimes they find the information they do get hard to understand.

*'Some of the patients had been told what they could and couldn't do. I didn't have information about the procedure and pain.'* Interviewed patient

*'I think I had all the information but it's such a lot of things to take in.'* Interviewed patient

**When to give patients information**

Most people who are anticipating treatment in hospital experience some anxiety before their admission, especially if they are going to have an operation and a general anaesthetic [**EXHIBIT 2, overleaf**]. Too often, talking to patients about pain and pain relief is left until after the operation when, from the patient's point of view, it would help to be told about it much earlier (Ref. 1). If nurses have the opportunity to meet patients before they are admitted – at a pre-operative assessment clinic, for example – this would be a good time to talk about pain and pain relief, to give the patient information in writing and to make clear that they can have the same information again on request. Good liaison between surgeons, anaesthetists and nurses can make sure that this happens without either missing anything out or any annoying repetition.

Where those kinds of opportunities for information-giving do not exist, it is important to take the earliest possible opportunity to talk to the patient about pain and the options for pain relief.

EXHIBIT 2

**Patients' worries about their anaesthetic and after-effects before their operation**

Many patients have concerns about the anaesthetic and how pain will be controlled.

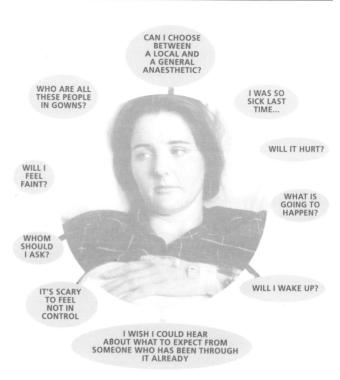

CAN I CHOOSE BETWEEN A LOCAL AND A GENERAL ANAESTHETIC?

WHO ARE ALL THESE PEOPLE IN GOWNS?

I WAS SO SICK LAST TIME...

WILL IT HURT?

WILL I FEEL FAINT?

WHAT IS GOING TO HAPPEN?

WHOM SHOULD I ASK?

IT'S SCARY TO FEEL NOT IN CONTROL

WILL I WAKE UP?

I WISH I COULD HEAR ABOUT WHAT TO EXPECT FROM SOMEONE WHO HAS BEEN THROUGH IT ALREADY

*Source: Audit Commission*
*(Ref. 1)*

## How to give information to patients

Patients like to have written information to back up what they have been told. They can read leaflets when they have the time to do so and they can use them to pass information on to their family and carers (Ref. 5). Professional staff and patients do not necessarily attach the same value to written information. In one study, for example, only 75per cent of nurses and 42 per cent of doctors – as compared with 90 per cent of patients – thought that an information sheet about post-operative pain was useful (Ref. 6).

Most patients who took part in the Audit Commission survey said that they had received information about pain verbally, but only one in five inpatients and one in three daycase patients had received information in writing. Almost all the patients who had been given written information found it either of some help or very helpful [TABLE 1].

TABLE 1

**Information about pain given to patients before their operation**

If you received written information, how helpful was it?

|  | Inpatients | Daycases |
| --- | --- | --- |
| Not at all helpful | 3% | 1% |
| Of some help | 58% | 42% |
| Very helpful | 39% | 57% |

*Source: Audit Commission survey*

9

**The content of information for patients**

There are good examples of written information already in existence. The Royal College of Nursing's Pain Forum has produced *Pain Control After Surgery: A Patient's Guide* (Ref. 7) with information on:

- pain and why it should be managed well;

- what patients can do before surgery and what their experience may be after;

- the importance of reporting pain;

- methods of pain relief;

- side effects;

- non-drug treatments, such as relaxation techniques and massage; and

- what to do at home.

If you want to write your own leaflet, find out first whether anyone else in your hospital has produced written information and what your colleagues in the multi-disciplinary team think of the proposal. They may already have designed and tested a leaflet that you can use as a framework for developing your own.

It is important to make sure that you collaborate and agree the content with colleagues from other disciplines, and that you include things that patients want to know as well as the things you think that they should know. You can do this only by including patients in the development of the leaflet, asking them their opinion about it and finding out whether it meets their needs.

Sometimes patients want to know more, but they do not know what to ask. It is useful to include prompts or questions that patients can ask and to emphasise how important it is that they let nurses know about their pain [BOX A]. You can also use the leaflet to illustrate a pain assessment tool and explain to patients how pain relief is administered.

BOX A

**The content of written information**

**You can encourage patients to ask questions such as:**

- will there be much pain after surgery?

- how long it is likely to last?

- who will be responsible for managing their pain relief?

- what pain relief methods will be used?

- will there be any unwanted effects?

**You can also use a leaflet to emphasise the positive effects of good pain relief and to remind patients that it is important for them to tell the doctor or nurse about:**

- previous experiences of pain and pain relief;

- other medicines they are taking; and

- any allergies that they know about.

### Daycase patients

Written information for daycase surgery patients should differ slightly from information for inpatients, in that the emphasis will necessarily be on helping patients to manage their own pain effectively. One hospital has produced booklets for day surgery patients (Ref. 8) that are relevant to the patient's surgery or condition. They cover:

- a brief explanation of what to expect on the day and during the post-operative period;

- advice on what to do if pain becomes severe; and

- information about a 24-hour helpline for patients to contact if their GP is not available.

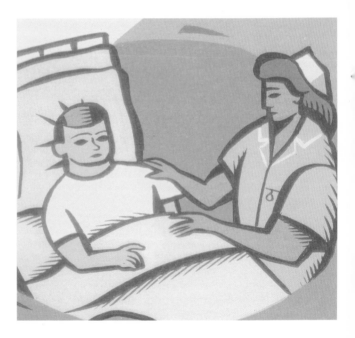

12

## Discharge home

Patients need to know what they can and cannot do once they are back at home, especially if they experience pain. If they are given analgesics to take home, they need to know when and how often to take them and what to do if they do not work. Most patients who took part in the survey were told what to do if they felt pain at home, but some patients were not told anything. Day surgery patients were more likely to be given information, and in writing, than inpatients [TABLE 2].

TABLE 2

Information about pain given to patients before their operation

Before leaving hospital, were you told what to do if you felt any pain at home?

|  | Inpatients | Daycases |
|---|---|---|
| Yes | 82% | 92% |
| No | 18% | 8% |

If 'yes', was any of this written information?

|  | Inpatients | Daycases |
|---|---|---|
| Yes | 32% | 61% |
| No | 68% | 39% |

*Source: Audit Commission survey*

**Making sure that the information reaches the patient**

Some hospitals produce good written information and/or buy in good written information from outside suppliers, but then lack the systems that they need to make sure that it reaches the right patient. It is very important to allocate responsibility for every stage in the distribution chain to named individuals. This means making sure the supplies of leaflets and booklets are always available in the hospital and in the right place, that someone monitors the supply and re-orders as necessary, and that there is an agreed and explicit plan for how the right leaflet will reach the right patient. It is important to make sure that the person responsible for handing the information to the patient understands its importance.

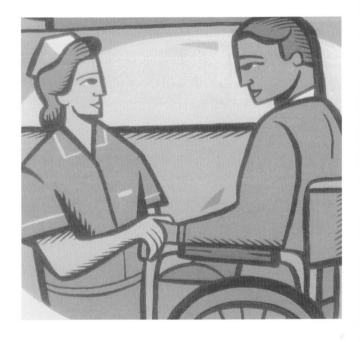

# What nurses can do

- Give patients a chance to ask questions and aim to give them information about whether they can expect to feel any pain; what to do if they are in pain; systems for administering pain relief; the options for pain relief; the possible side-effects of the different options available.

- Find out what patients are routinely told in outpatient and pre-screening clinics and make suggestions for using that opportunity to inform patients about pain relief.

- Find out whether the hospital has written information for patients about pain and pain relief. Check for yourself and ask patients on your ward whether the information is accessible; well-designed and laid out; and whether the print size is acceptable. Remember that many older patients suffer from visual impairment and you may be in an area with a large number of patients who do not speak or read English.

- Find out whether there is someone in the hospital with responsibility for producing written information; for ordering supplies and maintaining the stock; and for making sure that patients get the information that they need. If there is no written information about pain and pain relief available in the hospital, use leaflets already produced or organise a multi-disciplinary group to develop a leaflet or booklet. Do not forget to include patients in its development.

- Make someone on the ward responsible for the supply and distribution of written information.

- Have written information for patients to take home with them that describes what to do if they are in pain – if possible with a contact number; how and when to take any analgesics that they are given to take home and what to do if they experience side-effects; and what to take if they are in pain but have not been given any tablets.

- Make sure that the patient's GP is informed of the patient's discharge, including details of analgesics and any information that the patient has been given. Consider setting up an information 'hotline' for GPs and community nurses to obtain information about effective pain management.

# 3   Managing pain on the ward

Nurses are the one group of staff which is continually nearby and able to monitor patients' post-operative progress. They are the key to ensuring that patients remain free from pain after the initial prescription by the anaesthetist has worn off. If the original plan for analgesia turns out not to be working well, they are in a key position to spot this failure and seek advice on changing the programme.

There is also a wider clinical team involved in managing patients' pain, which includes doctors, physiotherapists and pharmacists. The team is more likely to succeed if all its members understand their role and responsibilities and there are agreed channels of communication between professionals.

The 1990 report by the Royal College of Surgeons and the College of Anaesthetists recommended the establishment of an acute pain team in every hospital (Ref. 2). Fifty-seven per cent of acute hospitals now have pain teams (Ref. 1) – the composition and responsibility of these teams vary but, typically, they are medically led – usually by a consultant anaesthetist – with the day-to-day responsibility for the practical work being undertaken by nurses.

In those hospitals with a pain team or a clinical nurse specialising in pain, it is usually possible for ward-based nurses to access advice on the management of individual patients with pain that is hard to control, patients with patient-controlled analgesia (PCA), and patients with epidurals. It is also more likely that ward nurses have someone to turn to for advice on how to measure pain, and on the guidelines that they should be working to.

Often the role of the specialist nurse on the acute pain team is defined as:

- liaison with nurses and doctors;

- education
  - running training days and seminars for nurses and junior doctors
  - disseminating data on the effectiveness of different analgesics and their side- effects; and

- audit
  - designing audit systems and collecting, analysing and reporting data.

In hospitals that do not have either a pain team or a clinical nurse specialist, the leadership for nurses on pain management needs to come from within the ward. Many wards (including wards in hospitals with an acute pain team) have found it useful to designate a lead nurse for pain from the ward team. Typically, that nurse's role is to make sure that the ward is working to the hospital's policies, standards, and guidelines on pain management. (If the hospital has not established policies and standards, ward nurses may bring this to the attention of senior nurses and the clinical directors for anaesthesia and surgery.) Sometimes wards decide to send the lead nurse on a special training course. On the ward, the lead nurse's role is to support and guide the other nurses in

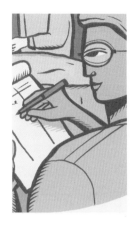

this area of care; to monitor the standard of documentation and to take the lead on auditing patients' pain.

Most nurses have experience of standard-setting and auditing practice against those standards. Where there is an acute pain team in the hospital, it should be the focus for developing standards across the hospital. But whether or not there is a pain team, it is important for individual wards to monitor their own effectiveness at managing patients' pain. Some wards use handover sessions for a team review of pain control care plans. Some wards and daycase units also arrange for one of the nurses to contact patients the day after their discharge as part of an audit on whether post-operative pain has been well-managed.

Pain management is constantly improving and it is important for nurses to learn about acute pain and pain relief and to keep up to date. Reading this booklet is a start and articles frequently appear in nursing journals. An ethos of good pain management can be generated on the ward by setting aside time for discussing and reviewing this area. Such occasions can be used for feedback on study days and other learning opportunities.

# What nurses can do

- If the hospital does not have an acute pain policy and a set of pain relief standards, ward nurses should bring this to the attention of senior nurses and the clinical directors of anaesthesia and surgery. The Royal College of Nursing's Pain Forum offers professional advice.

- In conjunction with the consultants responsible for their patients, clarify the roles and responsibilities of all members of the ward team including junior doctors, pharmacists and physiotherapists. Include responsibilities for communication and for audit.

- Consider asking one ward nurse to take the lead on pain. Know who is responsible for planning care for individual patients and how they should work with the lead nurse on pain if there is one.

# 4

# Delivering individualised patient care

*'Continuous, patient-centred care is central to the effective management of post-operative pain.'* (Ref. 2)

Patients vary considerably in the level of pain that they experience after the same operation and in how effectively different drugs and doses relieve their pain. Their methods of coping with pain also vary – some benefit most from controlling their own pain via PCA; others want clinical staff to bring pain relief at regular timed intervals; others prefer to keep their drug intake to a minimum (Ref. 9). If nurses can meet these individual needs and stop pain from breaking through, the patient-nurse relationship and the patient's entire hospital experience will benefit.

**Patient-centred care** is the only way to make sure that the individual pain relief needs of each patient are met. Remember that:

• two patients who have the same operation may need different pain relief; and

• the effective dose and the time taken for analgesics to work varies from patient to patient.

**Continuity of care** allows a small group of nurses to become familiar with how that patient experiences pain (Ref. 10). **Care plans** are the key to individualised care and continuity of care. Good record-keeping helps to improve communication. Care plans should include a standard method for recording the outcome of the assessment, making it easy to monitor pain and understand the effectiveness of analgesics for an individual patient. Plans should contain records of:

- pain levels;

- details of the pain relief administered;

- the effect of the pain relief, including side-effects; and

- what information has been given to the patient.

**Measuring pain**

The most important rules for managing pain are:

- 'pain is what the patient says it is'; and

- the patient's pain should be measured when the patient is moving as well as when the patient is at rest.

Many studies show that nurses assess patients' pain as being less acute than do the patients themselves (Ref. 4). Most general nursing assessment forms include space for recording the amount of pain that the patient experiences, but recording only what the patient says, 'a lot of pain' or 'not much pain', for example, is not helpful. To manage pain effectively, and especially to manage patients' pain over time, a more useful measure of what the patient feels – one that can be used once and used again – is needed.

A variety of reliable, tested pain assessment tools is available [BOX B] (Ref. 7). All the tools give the patient the responsibility for scoring his or her level of pain and their perception of the effects of analgesics. Some of the tools can be used in circumstances where the patient is unable to speak, or does not speak, English.

BOX 2

Pain assessment tools in common use

1. The pain thermometer used in the Burford nurse development unit

1   2   3   4   5   6   7   8   9   10

No pain at all   A little pain   Quite a lot of pain   A very bad pain   As much pain as I could possibly bear

2. A series of 'sad/smiley faces' is sometimes used for patients to indicate how they feel about their pain. These are translated into a simple score for recording on the care plan

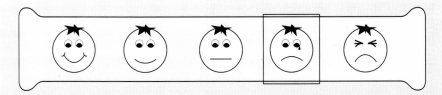

3. A series of descriptions that translate into a simple pain score can be used:

| | |
|---|---|
| No pain | 0 |
| Mild pain | 1 |
| Moderate pain | 2 |
| Severe pain | 3 |

*Source: Audit Commission site visits*

23

Self-assessment tools encourage consistency in pain measurement. In particular, they:

- give more accurate information on the level of pain;

- give information that helps to establish the pattern of pain;

- can be used to evaluate the effects of medication; and

- provide a framework for setting goals.

Some trusts also use flowcharts or 'algorithms' that set out the choices that can be made when managing an individual patient's pain. These are often based on the concept of an 'analgesic ladder', but they usually also include advice on what to do before and after giving medication.

**Modern analgesic methods**

Most modern pain management involves a combination of different types of pain control, and analgesics that are tailored to the needs of the individual patient and which change over time as the patient recovers from the operation. Sometimes anaesthetists insert local anaesthetic blocks that last for some hours after surgery; sometimes they give epidurals; and for some patients they prescribe drugs such as non-steroidal anti-inflammatory drugs (NSAIDs) and opioids. Here, we discuss briefly how these different methods affect the nurse's role in pain management. But the pharmacology of analgesics, and their side-effects, is a complex clinical subject that is beyond the scope of this booklet.

Drugs are not the only way of treating pain after surgery, but they usually play the major part in pain relief. Some non-pharmaceutical methods may be of benefit – for example, relaxation techniques and heat or cold treatments – and nurses are ideally placed to give advice about positioning, turning, and distraction activities such as listening to music. But there is no doubt that most patients will gain pain relief from drugs in addition to, or instead of, these techniques, as the scientific evidence about clinical effectiveness shows (Ref. 11).

Post-operative pain has typically been treated either by injection of a fixed dose of opioid every four hours, or 'as necessary'. But, today, the opportunity for individually tailored pain relief exists, because of:

- the wide variety of available drugs – ranging in strength from opioids, through NSAIDs, to minor analgesics such as paracetomol;

- the many forms of administration – including oral and suppository forms as well as injection, and continuous or patient-controlled infusion;

- changes in how often to give relief – for example, smaller doses of opioids given more frequently; and

- new ideas about 'balanced analgesia' – the combinations of drugs that can be given that interact to manage pain and unpleasant side-effects.

In the best instances pain management works very well, but the very strength of modern analgesia – the wide range of options available – leads to variation in what is used by anaesthetists, surgeons and wards within the same hospital (Ref. 1). A useful review of the scientific evidence about which analgesics are effective has recently been published (Ref. 11).

## Patient Controlled Analgesia (PCA)

PCA pumps allow the patient to self-administer small amounts of analgesic at frequent intervals, rather than receive large doses from a nurse that are hours apart. PCA is a safe and effective method of pain relief that is popular with patients if they have been carefully selected. But for some patients the bolus dose may not be large enough, the 'lockout period' may be too long, or they may become nauseous. PCA is suitable only for patients who are sufficiently alert to manage the pump. Patients who are considered suitable for PCA need to be fully informed.

*'It was a talisman. I felt safe with it in my hand. I didn't have to worry about the nurse not being there.'*
Interviewed patient

In the Audit Commission's survey of patients, there were some patients who had not been told that when they woke up after their operation they would be attached to a PCA pump [BOX C].

There will always be some patients who are concerned about taking responsibility for controlling their own pain and the nature of the drugs under their control – a recent survey confirmed that some patients lack understanding and receive inconsistent information about PCA (Ref. 12). It is always important for nurses to challenge myths about the dangers of addiction for patients who are prescribed opioids – whether they come from the patients or from their own professional colleagues:

*'They said push the button as much as you like. But you can get addicted can't you?'* Interviewed patient

BOX C

Some patients are not told about PCA before their operation

Of those patients who controlled their own pain, 86 per cent said that they were not told they would be doing this until they arrived on the ward and 37 per cent knew only when they awoke to find the PCA system in place. Almost one-quarter would have liked more information about the procedure.

Of those patients who were allocated to PCA, 63 per cent generally found it effective in controlling their pain, although one-third described it as only partly so. Three-quarters of patients experienced pain after PCA was stopped, and 68 per cent of these people subsequently experienced moderate to severe pain.

*Source: Audit Commission*

**Epidurals**

Epidural analgesia after major abdominal or thoracic surgery is becoming more common. However, it is more demanding of ward nurses' skills than PCA, and requires good training and support. To enable more patients to benefit from this form of pain relief, some hospitals will need to invest further in the training of ward nurses. At the moment, although 92 per cent of trusts report using epidurals in this way, patients are nursed on any of the surgical wards in only 40 per cent of them. In 30 per cent of these trusts, patients may be nursed only in certain designated wards, and in the remaining 30 per cent only in an intensive care or high dependency unit (Ref. 1).

# What nurses can do

- Make sure the ward has agreed protocols for acute pain management.

- Clarify responsibilities for care planning. Make sure that nurses are skilled in documenting care plans; that care plans include assessment of pain and a plan for its relief; and that the plan is evaluated and changed over time.

- Find out if the trust has flowcharts or 'algorithms' to help you to manage patients' pain.

- Use an objective measure for pain assessment and monitoring. Find out if there are assessment tools used in the hospital. It is good practice to use these consistently across wards in case either patients or staff are moved to other wards.

- Always have a supply of assessment forms available. Make sure that all ward staff are aware of the forms, why they are being used and how to use them.

- Make sure that patients are properly selected for PCA pumps, are fully informed well in advance of responsibility for the pain pump, and that their progress with the pump is monitored.

**BOX D**

**Good organisation and teamworking are the keys to ensuring pain-free patients after surgery.**

**For all patients**

- Purchasers should include specific standards about pain after surgery in their contracts.

- The trust's strategy should describe aims regarding pain control after surgery.

- Aims need to be translated into policies, standards, and guidelines for clinicians to follow; in-service training about what the trust expects, and audit of achievements are also essential.

- Resources should be earmarked to match agreed priorities (specialist staff, PCA and other pumps).

- Surgeons, anaesthetists, nurses and pain specialists must reach clear agreement about what has been delegated to whom.

- Consultant surgeons retain overall responsibility for the pain that their patients experience after surgery but anaesthetists also have a separate duty of care.

**For each individual patient**

- Make sure that someone is taking care of each step; the patient's named nurse is the most obvious person to check that this is happening.

cont. /

BOX D (cont.)

### ADMISSION
- Tell the patient what to expect
- Choice should involve the patient
- Back up with written information (eg, about PCA)
- Prescribe effectively

KEY STAFF: Admitting nurse, surgeon and/or anaesthetist

### RECOVERY ROOM
- Frequent pain scoring
- Pain controlled before leaving

As appropriate:
- Frequent, small analgesic doses
- Set up PCA

KEY STAFF: Recovery nurse, anaesthetist

### WARD/DAY UNIT
- Regular and frequent pain scoring (hourly in the first 24 hours) until no longer needed
- Listen to what the patient says
- Alter dose/drug vs. pain, nausea and respiratory rate scores

KEY STAFF: Ward/day nurse, surgical on-call, specialist advice

### HOME
- For day case procedures prescribe on basis of expected pain for operation, not on discharge pain score
- Back up with written information
- Liaise with GP, follow up by phone as appropriate

KEY STAFF: Ward/day nurse, anaesthetist

*Source: Audit Commission (Ref. 1), based on recommendations by pain specialists*

# Appendix 1
# When things work well–
# A case study

**Patients need accurate and full information**

The patient – Mrs Richards – received a letter telling her the date of her hysterectomy operation and asking her to attend a pre-assessment clinic. She was pleased to think that she would have an opportunity to find out about everything before actually going into hospital for the operation. The consultant had explained the operation to her at the outpatient clinic, but he had not mentioned pain, and she had not been given anything in writing. After an earlier operation she had experienced considerable pain, and she was concerned about the same thing happening again.

**Patients are often not confident enough to offer information unless asked**

At the pre-operative screening clinic Mrs Richards had her blood pressure tested, was weighed and asked about past illness and operations. She did not volunteer information about her previous experience of pain, nor did she express her worries.

**Giving written information in plenty of time is good practice**

However, the nurse invited her to talk about pain and told her that it would be possible to manage the pain using a 'pain pump'. The nurse also gave her a sheet of paper with information about the operation and the pain pump.

The information sheet told Mrs Richards that she had been selected as a suitable patient for this type of pain relief. It also emphasised that, although the drugs used in the pump are powerful, it is not possible to become

**Full written information can answer patients' questions and concerns**

addicted because there is a strict control on how much and how often it can be released into the body. It also contained information on why the PCA can be a good method of pain relief – that it avoids having to wait for the nurse to administer an injection or to give her tablets, and that provided the pain is under control before the PCA starts, the pain can be kept to acceptable levels.

**Anxiety can be avoided if staff take the time to explain what will happen**

After she was admitted to the ward and on the evening before her operation, Mrs Richards was visited by the anaesthetist who discussed the operation and the various methods of pain relief that were possible. He was followed by one of the ward nurses, who showed her the pain pump and the machine that it was attached to, and made sure that she understood what was to happen.

**Regular monitoring of the effectiveness of pain relief is good practice**

The anaesthetist began administering analgesia to Mrs Richards before she left the operating theatre and, once she had woken up, the nurse made sure that she was able to locate the button and press it as she had been instructed. It worked well and she felt both confident and in control. She continued to use the pump for a couple of days, with regular monitoring by the nurses. As her pain subsided, she was prescribed minor analgesia.

**Patients should be told what to expect and what to do when they go home**

Mrs Richards made a good recovery. She remained in hospital for several days and was prescribed painkillers to take home. A nurse gave her written information about when to stop taking the analgesia, what to do if she were to experience a worsening of her pain, and how to contact someone at the hospital if she was unable to reach her family doctor.

# Acknowledgements

The booklet was developed by Linda Jarrett, Jocelyn Cornwell and Dick Waite. It is one of a number of publications produced by an Audit Commission team that includes David Bawden and Lucy McCulloch. A full list of the hospitals in which patients, nurses, anaesthetists and other NHS staff were interviewed is given in the Audit Commission's report on anaesthesia and pain relief services in England and Wales, *Anaesthesia Under Examination* (Ref. 1). We are grateful to the many people who commented on a previous draft of this booklet. Responsibility for its contents and conclusions rests solely with the Audit Commission.

**References**

1. Audit Commission, *Anaesthesia Under Examination*, Audit Commission, 1997.

2. Working Party of the Commission on the Provision of Surgical Services, *Pain After Surgery*, Royal College of Surgeons and the College of Anaesthetists, London, 1990.

3. Burster S, Jarman B, Bosanquet N, Weston D, Erens R and Delbanco T L, 'National survey of hospital patients', *BMJ*, Vol. 309, pp1542-6, 1994.

4. Field L, 'Are nurses still underestimating patients' pain postoperatively?', *British Journal of Nursing*, Vol. 5, No. 13, 1996.

5.  Audit Commission, *What Seems To Be The Matter: Communication Between Hospitals and Patients*, Audit Commission/HMSO, London, 1993.

6.  Kuhn S, et al, 'Perceptions of pain relief after surgery', *BMJ*, Vol. 300, 30 June 1990.

7.  Royal College of Nursing's *Pain Forum, Pain Control After Surgery: A Patient's Guide*, RCN, undated.

8.  Hutson P, 'Pain following day surgery – are we doing enough?', *British Journal of Theatre Nursing*, Vol. 6, No. 7, October 1996.

9.  Copp L A, 'Pain coping', in Copp L A, (ed.), *Perspectives On Pain*; Recent Advances in Nursing, 11, Churchill Livingstone, Edinburgh, 1985.

10. Audit Commission, *Making Time for Patients: A Handbook for Ward Sisters*, Audit Commission/HMSO, London, 1992.

11. McQuay H, Moore A and Justins D, 'Treating acute pain in hospital', *BMJ*, Vol. 314, pp1531-5, 1997.

12. Coleman and Booker-Milburn, 'Audit of post-operative pain control', *Anaesthesia*, Vol. 51, pp1093-6, 1996.